Baby Sleep Training

*Top Tips and Secrets to Teach Your Baby
to Stop Crying and Sleep All Night - Better
Nights and Naps*

Introduction

Dear parents! So, your baby was born - this is the long-awaited native creation, a source of light and joy in the family.

In the first weeks of his life, night awakenings and feeding usually do not present any special difficulties for a young mother. She is overwhelmed with the happiness of the birth of her baby and is in a hurry to console him as soon as she hears a plaintive crying cry. She enjoys his intimacy and forgets about her own fatigue.

But over time, the latter accumulates, regular lack of sleep makes itself felt, getting up at night for young parents is becoming more difficult. And if a newborn baby usually falls asleep quickly and on his own, then the older he gets, the more difficult it is to lay him down.

Do not despair - these are temporary difficulties. Following the advice of this book, you can in just a few days teach your baby to quickly fall asleep in his crib on your own at any time convenient for you and sleep soundly all night.

Indeed, much depends on how much and when the child is sleeping: peace and quiet in the family, the health of the parents and their relationships with each other during this period, as well as the relationship between the parents and the child.

How to achieve this? Let's try it together. And if, as a result, peace and joy increase in your life, then it means that I wrote this book, not in vain.

Chapter 1: When and How Children Sleep

Speaking with young parents, I noticed that many of them are worried if their baby is sleeping enough. Usually, these fears are in vain - children sleep much less than we think. Sometimes a simple comparison with averages can open parents' eyes. So, my daughter, up to 2.5 years old, slept a total of 13 hours a day. And when she suddenly began to wake up earlier in the afternoon or in the evening she could not be put down, I was upset and wondered what had happened. Comparing the duration of her sleep with the average data obtained by interviewing numerous parents, I understood everything. It turns out that for 13 hours children usually sleep only up to six months of age! Then the duration of sleep gradually decreases and somewhere by 3 years reaches 11 hours. So, I was extremely lucky - my daughter slept for a long time longer than her peers!

Maybe this is the situation with you. Especially if the child sleeps irregularly, without a certain regimen, you may get the impression that he is "not sleeping at all," as some young parents complained during our conversations. The difference in hours is quite normal and may depend on many reasons, including how your baby spends the day, is accustomed to a clear regimen, does one fall asleep in his crib, does the child get enough parental love, and many other factors that will be discussed in this book.

For example, the need for sleep in newborn babies is very different. Some seem to sleep almost all the time, others not more than 14 in total, and in some cases even no more than 10 hours a day. This difference is rapidly decreasing, but the likelihood that a child who sleeps a lot from the very beginning and will continue to sleep more than other children of his age is quite high. Or vice versa - your baby is too curious and agile. Most likely, this will also have to be reconciled. Both that and another has, like everything in life, a reverse side of a coin. In addition, many children at school age are radically changing: those who are calm suddenly become overly mobile and noisy, and becomes lively and active, to the surprise of their parents.

On average, newborn babies sleep about 16 hours a day. They still do not distinguish night from day to day, and their sleep in the first three months is evenly distributed in "small portions" for night and day time. The older the baby becomes, the less he sleeps - his need for sleep is gradually reduced, and the world around him is becoming more interesting for him.

If in the first months of life a baby wakes up usually because he is hungry, then from the age of six months to a year the baby is already quite able to unlearn from night feedings. He has already understood the difference between daytime and nighttime and, if he is accustomed to it, he can easily sleep at night for 10 hours.

About why most children still wake up their parents at night and how to avoid this, I will tell in the next chapter. Together we will teach your baby to sleep more calmly, longer and at a time convenient for you.

Chapter 2: The Best Course Of Action for Sleep Problems: Prevention and Treatment

Why Do Children Wake up at Night?

The first step to solving any problem is to find out its causes. Therefore, in order to understand why your baby does not sleep well, you need to know some patterns of baby sleep.

Studying the sleep process in the laboratory with the help of electroencephalographs, scientists have found that sleep is not a homogeneous process, but consists of various phases, alternating in a certain sequence.

The first four phases are the various stages of the so-called slow, or deep, sleep with reduced activity of the body. After falling asleep, they succeed each other for 2-3 hours, and you yourself probably noticed that it was at this time that the child sleeps hardest. He is not disturbed by either light or noise, he does not even wake up if he is swaddled or carefully transferred, for example, from a stroller to a crib. This is the time when tired parents can finally relax and breathe a sigh of relief. If after an hour and a half after falling asleep, the baby starts tossing and turning in the crib, muttering something, doing sucking movements, etc. - this is not a cause for concern. Usually, this happens in a dream, during moments of incomplete awakening from a slow sleep, and then the baby sleeps quietly further.

After 2-3 hours, a slow sleep is replaced by a so-called fast sleep, or REM sleep (fast eye movements). It is called that because during it the eyeballs move quickly from side to side. With the transition to a fast sleep, the electroencephalogram of the sleeping person becomes the same as that of a waking person, his breathing and heartbeat increase, his temperature and pressure increase. It is at this time that your baby sees the most vivid and emotional dreams.

During REM sleep, a person is easy to wake. And just during the onset of this phase of sleep in the baby, his parents usually begin to prepare for night rest and make more noise than usual: they wash in the shower, brush their teeth with an electric brush or look into the room where the child is sleeping. If he wakes up, his parents are often annoyed, because most recently he slept so soundly that it was impossible to wake him up. (One young couple even complained in our conversations that their baby "seemed to wait specially until his parents settled down comfortably to immediately raise them to their feet again." Poor baby! No, people learn such things much later!)

Do not worry ahead of time if you woke up the baby during REM sleep: at the end of this phase he would wake up on his own. Because a short awakening after each phase of REM sleep before going to a slow sleep is a physiological pattern that is characteristic of both children and adults. And a similar phase change occurs up to seven times a night!

This means that absolutely all children wake up to seven times every night. Only some immediately fall asleep again, while others begin to cry, calling for help from their parents.

Common Mistakes Parents Make Trying to Get Their Children to Sleep

Why does this depend, you ask? Why does one child, waking up at night, fall asleep on his own, while another does not succeed without the help of his parents? As I already wrote, the phases of sensitive REM sleep with short-term awakening at the end are a kind of safety system for the body, which allows you to check whether everything around is in order, whether it is possible to sleep further. A small child, waking up at night, checks, for example, whether it is cold for him, whether he is hungry, whether it hurts anywhere, etc.

If the baby is tormented by intestinal colic (usually up to 4-5 months) or teething teeth (usually from 5-6 months), then it is at this time that they will interfere with his quiet sleep.

An incipient disease also often upsets children's sleep. A restless night may precede, for example, a cold or intestinal infection. Symptoms of many diseases appear for the first time just during a night's rest.

Frequent nocturnal awakenings can also be a reaction to vaccination. The underdeveloped immune system of the baby is in a state of anxiety, the body throws all its forces into the fight against an intruder. And if at the time of vaccination, the immune system was already busy fighting the incipient infection (still invisible to parents), now it has to fight on two fronts. She is overloaded with a new task, and the baby may have symptoms of an onset disease, which will also deprive him of night rest.

Maybe the child dreamed of something terrible. Indeed, at night, the children "process" the events of the day, which can be expressed in frightening dreams. If this happens occasionally and the baby quickly calms down and falls asleep when you appear, then there is no reason for concern. If your presence does not reassure the baby and it does not seem to notice you, then this may be a sign of the so-called night fright - a condition associated with incomplete awakening from a night's sleep. And the child, waking up at night, checks if everything is around as it was when he fell asleep.

And what turns out? He fell asleep on his warm, fragrant mother's shoulder, and wakes up in a cold, completely different smelling bed. Or he dozed off under the calming sway of a carriage, and now everything is motionless. Maybe he fell asleep, sucking on his mother's breast, a pacifier or a usual bottle of juice, but now they are gone ... And without them, the baby was not used to falling asleep. This means that it is urgent to "restore justice", and the baby cries loudly with all his infant strength, calling for help. His desperate cry cannot leave indifferent loving parents, and they, with difficulty rubbing their eyes, give the baby something that helps him fall asleep. That is, they again rocked, carried around the room, brought a bottle, sang songs, etc.

Having received the usual, the child quickly falls asleep again. But not for long: each new awakening ends with a new attempt to "restore justice." Moreover, the baby has already noticed that it is worth a little cry, and he will get everything he wants!

Tired parents are ready to do anything if only the baby fell asleep as soon as possible. Their fantasies literally have no limits. In addition to the most common methods of sedation, such as breasts, a dummy, a bottle, carrying on hands, motion sickness in a stroller, etc., many use unconventional methods. So, one father drove the baby for 20 minutes in the car, so that when he falls asleep, carefully put him in the crib. Many parents turn on the music, but there are those who start, say, a vacuum cleaner or a washing machine, because they noticed that uniform noise has a calming effect on the baby. A common way of laying is the presence of one of the parents in the baby's room until he falls asleep. Many pets a child, sing songs to him or just hold his hand. But one mother even climbed into the crib, so that the baby feels her intimacy. When the crib became small, this mother lay next to her on the floor (the crib was very low), resting her head on the pillow. Some babies like falling asleep to twisting their mother's hair, tickle her nose or do something like that. Often parents take the crying baby to their bed or, if the baby already knows how to get out of his crib, he climbs into the parents' bed himself.

No matter how convenient all these methods of momentary reassuring the child, they have one common drawback: the baby gets used to them and cannot fall asleep in a different way. Of course, if your baby, asleep in this way, sleeps peacefully all night, you have no reason to change anything. But usually, a child falling asleep only with the help of his parents needs her, day and evening, going to bed, and at night. For parents, this means a multiple night climb. In other words: having solved the problem at the moment, they create a lot of difficulties for themselves in the future.

To avoid them, there is only one way out: your child must learn to fall asleep on his own in his crib. If he learns to fall asleep in the day and evening, he can easily do this at night.

Of course, your baby will not immediately agree to give up pleasant and convenient habits for him. But the efforts made will pay off because a good night's sleep is important first of all for the baby. In addition, children are happy when their parents are calm, and parents are calm when they get enough sleep at night...

Getting Your Baby to Fall Asleep According to Her Internal Clock Naturally

Too many parents overestimate the child's need for sleep. And when the baby suddenly wakes up at night and for a long time (longer than an hour) cannot fall asleep, when he wants to play in the middle of the night or demands the attention of his parents in some other form, they are often at a loss.

In fact, everything is very simple - your child in total sleeps too much. And since the baby's sleep is not optimally distributed during the day, it turns out to be enough sleep just at the moment when it's the least convenient for you - in the middle of the night. He simply has a disturbed, shifted rhythm of sleep and wakefulness, which is very easy to change.

First, you need to calculate how many hours a day the child really sleeps. This is his daily need for sleep. The number of hours a baby spends in his crib needs to be reduced to this figure.

Now it remains only to distribute the child's hours of sleep at a time convenient for you. For example, if he sleeps twice during the day, then most likely, now he needs only one, then the night's sleep will become calmer. The only, but too long daytime sleep is to "shorten", that is, to wake the baby earlier. Or, if it's more convenient for you, you can wake the child earlier in the morning. Another possibility is to lay the baby later in the evening. Whichever option you choose, one thing is important - that the time spent by the child in the crib does not in total exceed the baby's calculated need for sleep.

And the sequence in your actions is also important because, in order to get used to the new regime, the baby needs time (usually no more than a week). Of course, it's a pity to wake a baby sleeping peacefully, especially in the morning, when parents still want to sleep. But tolerate only a week, and you will no longer need to wake the baby - he will wake up himself in due time. Well, for parents, getting up earlier in the morning is nevertheless more pleasant than "walking" in the middle of the night, isn't it?

Obstacles for Working Moms and Children with Sleep Issues

Well, there are many ways to help a baby fall asleep. But why, you ask, does one baby need help with this, and the other, it seems, is calm from birth, sleeps peacefully or, waking up, lies calmly in his crib?

To understand the phenomenon of calm children, look at their mothers. Ask them about how the pregnancy went, about their attitude to life, relationships with a partner, etc. You will find that calm children almost always have calm mothers!!! Because nothing affects the physical, mental and emotional development of the baby so much as the state of a person who is carrying it under the heart, breastfeeding and caring for the baby day and night! The mother's energy, health, and mental state, her joys and sorrows, worries and fears are transferred to the child and either give him peace and confidence or deprive them. Therefore, if you want your baby to be calm, take care of yourself first!

Already during maternal pregnancy, a tiny creature hears, feels and perceives everything that happens around it. Everything that happens in the mother's body is directly transmitted to the baby through the umbilical cord. Her mental state, however, reaches the crumb as through invisible waves and fills with joy or fear, calm or nervous tension. If a pregnant woman gets enough sleep, walks a lot, eats well and - most importantly - enjoys life and upcoming motherhood, then the chances that the baby will be born calm are much greater than if she eats somehow, gets tired, nervous and quarrels with her husband. So, scientists at the Center for the Study of the Health of Children and Adolescents at the University of Bristol (UK) found that prolonged depression in mothers during pregnancy, as well as in the first months after birth, entails 50% of cases of impaired development and behavior of infants!

Parental characteristics also influence the establishment of consolidated sleep as they are associated with certain sleeping habits or practices. Anxious, overprotective, depressed or insecure mothers in their attachment history would tend to have more children with sleep problems than other mothers. For example, studies have shown that depressive mothers influence the consolidation of the child's sleep. This relationship could be due to a modification of maternal behaviors (overprotection) thus hindering the child's learning about his autonomy to sleep.

You may be stressed at work and cannot wait to see the nanny out when you arrive. However, if you want your baby to be calm, be calm yourself! Laugh, enjoy life, and then your child will also prefer the joy of life to cry and whims.

Chapter 3: Navigating the Tricky Newborn Phase Like A Pro

The fact that a clear regimen greatly facilitates caring for a child, we know from childhood. In the last chapter, we also found out that the regimen helps the baby sleep better because, by the age of 4-6 months, each baby develops an "internal clock" due to which his body switches to sleep at the usual time and the baby falls asleep better and faster. Children who are accustomed to sleeping in the afternoon haphazardly, with the transition to a clear regimen, sleep longer. And mom has regular, pre-planned "oases" of free time. I repeat that it will be wise if she uses this time to relax, because you can't do all the work, and fatigue tends to accumulate. Using free time for herself, mom will indirectly take care of the baby, because for him there is nothing better than calm, rested parents!

Regular feeding is also very important - they contribute to the baby's feeling of hunger at a certain time. Knowing when the baby is sleeping and when eating, you can plan your day: go somewhere, make an appointment or do something that is possible only at a specific, prefixed time. Of course, from plans that are not comparable with the time of the baby's sleep, you will have to refuse at first. But when the baby gets used to the regime and completely reorganizes on it (usually this happens within two to three weeks), it will be possible to make exceptions.

In the West, and in recent times more and more often with us, one can hear supporters of regimeless care of a child when he sleeps and does not eat by the clock, but when he wants to. Doctors supporting this method believe that this best meets the needs of the baby in the first time of his life and favorably affects his development. They also argue that the rhythm forms over time by itself, without parental intervention.

And what happens in practice? According to the results of my surveys, out of ten parents who used this method, nine later regretted it. Only in one case out of ten the baby gradually independently reorganized into a certain mode acceptable for parents. In other families, non-regime care led to chaos in the passage of the day and, as a consequence, fatigue, and discontent of parents. They could not plan their day, because they never knew when the baby would fall asleep. The kids, who slept for a long time during the day, were rested and active at night. And some even "mixed up night and day," and parents could not sleep a wink almost the whole night. Irregular feeding led to the fact that when the baby cried, the parents did not know if he was hungry or crying for another reason. Breastfeeding mothers, in this case, were especially often soothing babies, giving them breasts. Whether the children were really hungry will always remain a mystery, but the fact that they were comfortable and calm on their mother's breasts is a fact, therefore the kids, at least because of this, did not want to give up this pleasant habit for a long time. As a result, mothers complained that all day they only knew that they were feeding the baby and that they had no time for anything else. And some of the children who received in this way too much milk for a still very small stomach constantly vomited. And even in this case, a rare caring mother guessed that the baby is absolutely healthy, he just eats too often.

The moral of this is that a clear daily routine is important not only for parents but also for the kids themselves. Moreover, we already know that a child is healthy and calm only if his parents are calm and happy...

When to Start Sleep Training

So, when should the regime start? Of course, the sooner the better. If in the first weeks of his life the baby still lives in its own uncontrollable rhythm, then in 1.5-2 months he is quite able to slowly begin to adapt to the outside world and to a convenient time for you to feed and sleep. This does not mean that he should scream, waiting for the next feeding. Everything needs to be done gradually, increasing, for example, a little between the feedings and calming the baby until the right time by other means.

3-4-hour pauses between meals will most likely meet your baby's needs and will be acceptable to you. Of course, pauses can be shorter or longer, they can be slightly different during the day, depending on when and how much the child sleeps, and on your needs. The main thing for the "internal hours" of the baby is that the feeding takes place every day at about the same time.

Of course, sleep should also be regular. At the age of 1.5 months, you can try the "two-hour method" offered by German doctors: from the moment the baby wakes up to the moment when you put him back in the crib, two hours should pass. Only in the evening is it worthwhile from the very beginning to adhere to a certain, convenient for you laying time, even if the baby has to spend more than two hours without sleep for this. But, tired, this time he will sleep longer, which will usher in the habit of a long night's sleep.

Short-circuit for months, when a child already has three "quiet hours" a day, it makes sense to enter a certain time for daytime sleep. Decide in advance when it is more convenient for you to lay your baby, and stick to this time every day. If the baby falls asleep on the go, try not to let him fall asleep. This will require strength from you, but after a maximum of a week your baby will get used to the new regime and will sleep at the time you set, and you can start planning your day. In the evening, still, put the baby at the same time.

If the baby does not sleep well at night, do not give him the opportunity to sleep too long during the day. One and a half to two hours of daytime sleep at a time is enough for a child. Do not be afraid to wake him at first when the time is up - in a few days he will get used to a new rhythm and will wake up himself. It is especially important that the baby does not sleep too long in the afternoon.

Prolonged wakefulness at the end of the day will help him sleep better at night. In addition, too long a "quiet hour" makes it difficult to comply with the regime: the child who has been sleeping for a long time during the day is difficult to lay down next time. When you finally succeeded, it turns out that time has moved and the whole regime is violated...

There are, of course, children who themselves sleep much less during the day, sometimes no longer than half an hour at a time. You probably have to put up with it. Usually, children who sleep little at all do not sleep for long. But, as already mentioned, even these babies can learn to sleep an hour longer if they fall asleep according to the regimen and on their own in their crib.

To teach a baby to fall asleep in a crib without the help of parents is from the very beginning. To do this, regularly put him before bedtime in the crib (if he is still small and cannot sleep alone, then at least for a short time, so that the baby slowly gets used to this feeling, and does not end up in the crib only after he has comfortably fallen asleep at mom or dads shoulder). According to experience, babies aged 2-3 months are the easiest to learn to fall asleep on their own.

To make a schedule that is convenient for you and your child, calculate how many hours a day your baby sleeps at the moment, how many of them he is able to sleep at night and how much remains respectively, for daytime sleep. Now you only need to determine when it is most convenient for you to lay the baby in the evening, as well as for how many receptions and at what time he will sleep during the day.

For example, the regime of a three - month - old baby sleeping three more times a day can look like this: night sleep from 21:00 to 6:00, daytime sleep from 9:00 to 11:00, from 13:00 to 14:30 and from 16:30 to 18:00.

Starting from the age of six months, two "quiet hours" a day are enough for a baby. So, he could sleep at night from 21:00 to 7:00, and during the day from 10:30 to 12:00 and from 15:30 to 17:00. (The waking time before bedtime should be the longest and last at least 4 hours).

And in a year and a half, most children switch to single daytime sleep, and you can put your baby, for example, at night from 21:00 to 7:00 and in the afternoon from 13:00 to 15:00.

The older the child, the easier it is for him to adapt to the mode you set. But in any case, to get used to the new daily routine, the baby will need time (up to three weeks), which will pay off in the future.

Having prepared a daily routine for the child, do not forget to regularly review it, adapting the regimen to the age and changing needs of the baby!

Why Both Night Sleep and Day Sleep Are Important?

Why not scrap daytime sleep, you may think? At least, say, as the baby grows a bit? Well, daytime sleep has a positive effect on many factors in the development of the baby. First of all, daytime sleep, however, like nighttime, promotes the development of growth hormone. Oddly enough, but it is in a dream that children grow faster.

One of the tasks of daytime sleep is to protect the child's nervous system. During sleep, the child's brain is resting, which helps to cope with the large-scale amount of information that is especially characteristic of the first years of life.

Thus, all "vital material" is processed by the child's brain in small portions, shared by daytime sleep.

In addition, today a direct relationship between sleep and baby activity has been proven. So, if a child does not receive the necessary hours of sleep at intervals of day and night, he becomes nervous and irritable, and sometimes even foci of uncontrollable impulsiveness and even aggression arise. Also, day and night sleep can have a positive effect on the work of certain organs, for example, the intestines and bile ducts.

Sleeping Late, Waking Early: Handling Nap-Resistant Kids

It may happen that you are quite happy with your baby's daytime sleep, but you won't be able to put him in the evening for a long time, or, on the contrary, he rises in the morning with no light. Usually, these problems are easily solved by introducing a clear, convenient daily routine for you, as described above. If you have entered the regimen, but the child still maintains his habit of getting up early or going to bed late, this may have several reasons.

Firstly, among both adults and children, pronounced "owls" and "larks" are found. Usually, this is inherited, and retraining such a child to adhere to a different sleep regimen is almost impossible (and undesirable for his health). But do not despair ahead of time - in most cases, late falling asleep or early awakening are due to completely different reasons.

The reason may be, for example, because in the daily routine you took the baby for a night's sleep for too long. After 6 months, children, no matter how much they sleep during the day, rarely sleep at night for longer than 10-11 hours.

Therefore, if you put the baby in the evening too early (for example, at 7 o'clock in the evening), it will not be at all surprising that he will rise in the morning before you (perhaps already at 5 o'clock in the morning). Lay him down in the evening later, and if it is not a neon "early bird", it will soon please you in the morning with a later awakening.

And if you allow your child to sleep for too long in the morning or in the afternoon, then most likely he is not tired enough in the evening and therefore cannot sleep for a long time. Wake him at a convenient time for you in the morning or afternoon, and soon fatigue will win - the baby will voluntarily go to bed earlier in the evening.

Of course, he will need time to get used to the new regime, and this time will require special understanding and patience on the part of his parents. But bear the baby's whims for two weeks, and his night's sleep will move in the right direction, his "internal clock" will switch to a new rhythm.

Another possible mistake in the daily routine is the improper time of the first or last day's sleep. Babies who go to bed too early in the morning often wake up very early in the morning and then fill up in the afternoon. In this case, move the first "quiet hour" to a later time. If your baby sleeps twice during the day, then the first time it should be laid no earlier than 2.5 hours after morning awakening. And if he sleeps only once during the day, then put him to bed not earlier than noon.

Children sleeping too late in the afternoon are usually difficult to put in the evening. Plan your last night's sleep so that the baby is awake for at least 3-4 hours before a night's sleep. A child who is tired at the end of the day will fall asleep faster and easier in the evening at an earlier time.

A baby may wake up early either due to early morning feeding or because one of the family members rises early. If the baby is used to the first feeding at five in the morning, then an empty stomach will regularly wake him up at this time. Try to delay the time of morning feeding, calming the baby in other ways. After some time, he will break the habit of eating "early in the morning" and, probably, will sleep longer in the morning.

In the morning hours the baby sleeps especially sensitively, the phases of REM sleep (with a short awakening at the end) become more frequent in the morning. And since the child had already practically slept by this time, it becomes more difficult for him to fall asleep after each awakening. If someone has to get up early in the family, he can finally wake up the baby with any rustle, even if he tries very hard not to make noise, walk on tiptoe.

In this case, you can only lay the baby earlier in the evening to get enough sleep at least in the evening. And in the morning, if you are not in a hurry, you can take the baby to your bed. A cozy start to the day and a portion of tenderness in advance will charge you both with energy for the whole day.

One of the reasons that a child is difficult to lay in the evening may be his habit of falling asleep only in your presence or in your arms. Noticing that he does not have time to close his eyes, as you carefully try to put him into the crib or leave the room, the next time the baby will carefully monitor you so as not to miss this moment. "If I fall asleep, I will remain alone in the crib (or room)," his experience will tell the baby. And the child will, by all means, resist fatigue. What to do? There is only one way out - to teach him to fall asleep without your help, alone in his crib (how to do this will be discussed in the next chapter).

If the baby, who easily fell asleep in the evening at the appointed time, suddenly becomes unstoppable, the reason may be that he simply became older and therefore did not sleep as long as before. Maybe it's time to review the regimen, reducing the overall duration of the baby's sleep.

To do this, you can reduce the number of "quiet hours" or their duration. If the baby slept once during the day, then you can abandon daytime sleep altogether. And if the daytime pause and evening rest are equally important to you, you just have to wake the baby earlier in the morning until he is rebuilt and wakes up earlier himself.

For older children, who don't even sleep during the day, and in the evening try to delay their sleep time with hundreds of different desires and ideas (not because they want to make you angry, but because they are simply not tired enough), it's quite possible to allow to go to bed an hour later. The condition is that they must spend this hour playing a quiet game in their room. At this time, it is allowed to read (or just view) books, play, listen to music or a fairy tale, but not allowed to make noise, jump, run or leave the room unnecessarily. Arrange with the baby that in an hour you will come to his room to turn off the light and wish him goodnight. If he wants this, you can tell him a bedtime story (but only one, so that this does not become a new way of delaying time). After this, the child should stay in bed. Only in this case will he be again allowed to play before bed the next day.

Of course, such an arrangement makes sense only when the child already really needs less sleep and can easily get up at the appointed time in the morning. If not, then wait until the hour of a quiet game before bedtime becomes a habit and the baby then goes to bed voluntarily, and then quietly move the start of the game to an earlier time, so that the child eventually ends up in bed.

The problem with evening falling asleep on certain days may be related to how the baby spent that day or evening before going to bed.

If an older, active, full of impressions day gets tired of the older children, and then they sleep better, then the babies are still not able to cope with the large stream of impressions falling on them and are quickly overexcited. They begin to act up, cry, and in this state, it is difficult for them to fall asleep. (After all, you know by yourself: when the head is full of impressions and experiences, it's even difficult for us adults to disconnect, and sometimes we cannot close our eyes for a long time). Think about whether too many events are happening in your child's life in the first months. Try to have a calmer day. It is very possible that this will help the baby fall asleep faster and sleep better at night.

Older children are often difficult to put to bed because of an overly moving evening. Having run up, having jumped, having ridiculed a lot, they cannot fall asleep for a long time. Children need time to calm down and switch to sleep. Therefore, the last hour or two before bedtime must necessarily take place in a calm atmosphere. Refuse outdoor games in the evening, guests and everything that can excite a child. Dim the light, try to speak quietly, let the baby understand that a calm time of day is coming.

Some children fall asleep better after an evening swim. Maybe this will help your child.

And be sure to talk with the baby as much as possible. Explain to him that the day is coming to an end and you need to prepare for bed. Talk again about the most important and interesting events of the past day ("today you and I walked in the forest", "our grandmother was visiting, she was very glad to see you," etc.). Then tell us what your plans are for tomorrow ("tomorrow, when you wake up and eat, we will go to the store to buy you new pants."). In the end, tell the baby that he should now sleep in order to gain strength for a new, interesting, full of pleasant surprises day. Even a baby who does not yet understand your words will feel your love in this way and will fall asleep with a calm confidence that it will be so tomorrow. And the older kid will hasten to fall asleep so that this interesting tomorrow will come soon.

Effective Strategies for Naps

So, relax, yes, but how? There are many techniques. Here is a list proposed by Dr. Koa Whittingham and Pamela Douglas, choose those that tempt you, some can be done with your baby during breastfeeding or a walk. But they all serve the same goal – they will get even the most troublesome kids get ready for a nap session.

1. Breast-feed
2. A hot bath
3. Cuddle baby
4. Listen to relaxing music
5. Healthy touch (massage baby with soothing baby-friendly oils)
6. Sucking on a pacifier, toy or thumb
7. Hugs
8. Skin-to-skin contact
9. The rocking of the stroller

I guess I'm not teaching you anything, however, try combining these activities and you will find relaxing activities for you and your baby. Try to make the famous routine relaxing for you too.

Chapter 4: How to Teach a Child to Fall Asleep Independently

Refusals to Go to Bed

So, dear parents, you have already found out that one of the most important prerequisites for a calm and prolonged night sleep of the baby is the ability to fall asleep independently in his crib. But how to teach him to do this?

Why does even a very tired baby falling asleep in your arms begin to cry when she suddenly finds herself in a crib? And why does an older child rarely go to sleep himself and sometimes fall asleep right during the game, one can say, against his will?

1. Each baby craves most of all the closeness of her parents. To be alone in bed means for him to part with his parents, not to feel any more of their calming intimacy and native warmth. Of course, a rare baby will agree to this without protest,

especially if he is spoiled by parental attention during the day and "does not get away from it."

2. Often, the baby falls asleep while breastfeeding or in her mother's arms. Noticing once that he should fall asleep, as his mother tries to carefully transfer him to the crib, the baby will next time struggle to resist sleep so as not to miss this moment. Asleep, he will sleep very sensitively. Feeling how you put him in the crib, he will immediately wake up and express his disagreement with a loud cry. Try to fall asleep yourself if you know, for example, that as soon as you close your eyes, someone will steal your blanket...

3. Maybe the baby happened to wake up at night in the crib with a wet, frozen, hungry or frightening nightmare. He felt lonely and forgotten, and he had to wait longer for the arrival of his mother than it was in the afternoon. After such an experience, the baby may experience a subconscious fear of going to bed and protest, being alone in his crib.

4. Very often, the baby we are trying to put to bed is just not tired enough.

5. For an older child, going to bed means parting with some interesting activity, ending the game, saying goodbye to the guests sitting in the next room, etc.

6. Knowing that parents or older brothers and sisters have not yet gone to bed, the baby does not want to accept this "injustice".

7. Some children are afraid of the dark.

8. Sometimes children do not want to go to bed simply because we spoiled them. The child uses the evening persuasion of parents to stretch time, or they serve as an occasion for self-affirmation.

Sometimes, however, it may turn out that helping your baby fall asleep is easier than you thought. So, fearful children can be reassured by a night light or an open door to the nursery, while older children fall asleep more willingly if they are allowed to go to bed an hour later.

How to Teach a Baby to Fall Asleep from the Very Beginning

To teach a baby to fall asleep without the help of parents and without any auxiliary means is possible at any age. But babies aged 1.5 to 3 months are most easily used to this. Therefore, it is better to start with accustoming gradually from birth, until the child is still accustomed to various kinds of unfavorable rituals, from which it is then not so easy to wean them. If such habits have already developed, parents will need a little more patience, because the baby is unlikely to abandon them voluntarily. But even in this case, the problem is completely solvable, and most likely it will take no more than a week to solve it!

1. In order to teach an infant to fall asleep independently, it is necessary from the very beginning to put him alone in the crib as often as possible, nevertheless remaining close to him. If you carry the baby in your arms all day or rock him in the carriage during the day, then, being alone in a fixed bed, he will feel insecure. This feeling will be unusual for the baby, and he is unlikely to be

able to sleep peacefully. Accustomed to the crib, the baby feels calm there, and in the usual environment, any child falls asleep better.

2. Putting one baby in a bed does not mean leaving him there for a long time, especially if he is crying. No, of course, the crying child needs to be reassured. But as soon as he stopped crying, do not carry him on your hands. Lay him again so that he sees you or hears your voice. Talk to him, sing to him, but leave him in the crib so that he gradually gets used to it. Among other things, the child will learn how to deal with himself in this way: look at his pens or play with them, look around, listen to the sounds around him, etc. Well, you yourself will have time to do more things that you wouldn't have time to do if the baby was in your arms all the time.

3. If the baby first falls asleep only on your chest, that's okay. No need to wake him up. To begin with, it will be sufficient if he gets used to his crib while awake. When he appears in a mode with a certain sleep time, you need to gradually begin to separate food and sleep. It is better to feed those

who like to fall asleep on their chest or with a bottle when they wake up, or at least some time before bedtime. And by the time the baby usually falls asleep, you need to put him alone in the crib. By this time, he was already tired and his "internal clock" switched to sleep, so it will be easier for him to fall asleep without your help.

4. At first, it is not necessary to put the baby alone in the bed before bed every time. You can start one or two times a day, at the same time when the baby, in your experience, falls asleep the easiest. For most children, this is evening, but there are children who fall asleep faster in the morning or afternoon. The main thing is that you and the baby feel that falling asleep independently is, in principle, possible. Then it will become a habit - it is only a matter of time.

5. And what if you put a baby in bed before bed and he begins to cry bitterly? Try to calm him down first without picking up. Stroke him, sing a song, talk to him, tell how you love him. Explain that it is time to sleep in order to gain new strength, that you

are near and will protect the baby while he sleeps. If the baby is still crying, hold him in your arms. But as soon as he calms down, put him back in the crib. Crying again - try to calm him down again, without picking up, and only then, if all is in vain, take the baby from the crib. Maybe he is still too small and it is worth waiting a couple of weeks, then again carefully starting to accustom him to falling asleep again. And from six months of age, it is already possible to move on to the method of Dr. Ferber, which will be presented later, in the section "If the child does not want to go to bed alone."

6. Some babies are helped to fall asleep with a pacifier. But as soon as the baby is fast asleep, carefully remove the nipple from his mouth, otherwise he will wake up when he loses it in his sleep. And if the baby, waking up at night, is looking for a pacifier and crying, then it can become effective help only when he learns to find it himself.

7. Infants in the first months of life sleep better if they rest against the top of their heads in a rolled

diaper, pillow or back of the crib protected by a blanket. It reminds them of a sensation in the womb. (My daughter loved this feeling even at an older age. I always covered the upper headboard with a blanket, and my daughter laid on the very top of the pillow to rest her head against it.)

8. You can also harder to swaddle the baby before bedtime, which also reminds him of the tightness before birth. And when the baby becomes older, he can be helped by a sleeping bag or mother's shirt, knotted from below.

9. Mom's smell generally has a calming effect on babies, and you can just put something from your mother's (worn) clothes next to the baby's head.

10. But do not forget that the main condition for the child to fall asleep on his own is the correctly chosen laying time. The kid must really get tired, otherwise attempts to lay him will not succeed. The easiest way for you to succeed if you

have already entered a strict daily routine. In this case, you know in advance when the "internal clock" of the child will switch to sleep. If not, you will have to rely on your intuition and experience. A tired baby begins to yawn, rub his eyes or be naughty for no reason. Try to guess the most successful moment when his eyes already close by themselves to put him alone in the crib.

Rituals of Falling Asleep - the Step-By-Step Baby Sleep Training Methods and How to Teach Your Baby to Fall Asleep Within 10 Minutes Based on the Baby's Age

We have already said that you will greatly facilitate the baby falling asleep if you make sure that his last hour before bedtime passes in a calm, familiar, full of love atmosphere. This is the time of transition from the active part of the day to calm, from new impressions to familiar comfort, from noise and outdoor games to peace and quiet...

The introduction of the so-called ritual of falling asleep - the actions that are repeated daily in a certain sequence and develop a kind of conditioned reflex for the baby - will help the child to calm down and tune in to sleep. Elements of such a ritual can be, for example, bathing, massage, swaddling, putting on pajamas, brushing teeth, reading a fairy tale, your favorite lullaby, doll or soft toy, "going to bed" with the baby, etc. And, of course, the tenderness of the parents and my mother's favorite voice, which will be remembered by the baby all his life!

It probably happened to you that some smell or taste suddenly evoked pictures from your childhood in your memory or some detail in clothes reminded of a specific person. So, in children who are accustomed to a certain evening ritual, a familiar melody or favorite toy in the crib will soon begin to be associated with sleep. And the intimacy and love of parents at this time will fill the baby's soul with the confidence that he is desired and loved, and with this confidence, it will be much easier for the baby to fall asleep alone.

For children who are accustomed to falling asleep only with the help of various kinds of auxiliary means (bottle, etc.), the introduction of the ritual of falling asleep will help to abandon them. The new ritual, as it were, will replace the old habit and facilitate the transition to the moment when the baby is alone in her crib.

Rituals of falling asleep are important for both infants and older children, so their content should be changed in accordance with the age and needs of the child.

1. In the first year of the baby's life, the routine part of the ritual (preparation for bed) is still closely intertwined with parental tenderness, affectionate words, and touches. Bathing, swaddling or changing clothes in the evening, you can stroke him, massage him, sing songs, talk about the past and the new day. Do not forget to do this every day in the same sequence so that the baby knows in advance what will happen next. Only in this case, these actions will become for the child a ritual and a signal for sleep. When laying the baby in the crib, you must say the same phrase, which will become familiar to him, for example: "now it's time to sleep to gain strength for a new day" (or some other that will let the baby understand that the time has come to sleep). Curling the curtains, turning off the lights (turning

on the children's nightlight) and a gentle kiss with the words: "Goodnight, son (daughter)!" I love you very much! "- will be the final point ritual, after which you must leave the room. And act confidently, because, having felt the uncertainty in your actions or your voice, the baby will surely try to keep you offended by crying. (What to do if the child is crying, we will talk in the section "If the child does not want to go to bed alone (Ferber method)").

2. In order to track whether the baby has fallen asleep, it is very convenient to have such an invention as a baby monitor. Turning it on, you can safely move around the house, and not stand on tiptoe at the door, listening to every rustle behind it.

3. For older children, the routine preparation for bedtime can be reduced to the required minimum, but the cozy part with mom or dad in the children's room should be slightly stretched. This is the time when the baby enjoys the undivided attention of his parents - half an hour,

belonging to him alone. You can sit the child on your lap, read a book to him or simply look at the pictures together, calling out loud what is depicted on them. Or maybe you will sing to the baby or tell him a good story. Many people and in adulthood remember mother's tales and lullabies. Or you can quietly turn on the cassette and swing with the child, for example, in a rocking chair. If the baby is used to falling asleep with his favorite toy, you can engage her in the evening ritual. Let the bunny, bear or doll then tell the child that it is time to go to bed and ask if he will allow them to sleep with him today. Unleash your imagination in these minutes. But remember that all your actions should become a habit for the baby and be repeated day after day, even if you find it boring. Only in this case, cozy minutes before bedtime will be associated with the child falling asleep.

4. When choosing an evening ritual, it is very important to determine its time frame in advance and warn the baby about them. If you don't do this, the child will not want to stop and will try to stretch out a pleasant occupation with all his might ("one more story, mother, well, please, ah …"). The easiest way is to draw the border immediately and

agree with the baby that you will read to him, for example, only one story or only one children's book. You can show the clock in the room and say that you will read until this hand reaches this figure. This will seem logical even to a kid who doesn't know the numbers. Having defined boundaries, remain firm and do not violate them even as an exception. Feeling the weakness, the child will try to use it to delay the time of sleep. You will become impatient. The baby, having felt this, he will begin to be capricious, and the whole ritual will no longer have the desired effect.

5. The final point of the ritual for older children is the same as for small children (drawn curtains, turned off lights, a gentle kiss with gentle words for the night). If you used a clock to determine the time frame, now is just the right moment to point your child at it. For example, with the words: "Well, look - the small arrow has already reached the number "seven"," you put away books with toys and put the baby in the crib.

All the elements of the ritual in this chapter are just examples. You can use them or come up with your own, unique. After all, you know your child better than others - what he loves, what he needs, what calms him.

1. For example, bathing has a calming effect on most children, but there are those that it excites. In addition, daily contact with water can cause irritation to sensitive baby skin, and an allergic reaction may occur to the most neutral baby shampoo if used daily. Strong-smelling shampoos sometimes have an exciting effect, but special soothing essential oils can help your baby fall asleep, unless, of course, he is allergic to them.

2. Kids love bedtime massage very much. To do this, it is not necessary to go to special courses and learn certain techniques (although this can be useful). Cautious, affectionate stroking along the entire body of the baby, from head to toe, he will surely like it. Rely on your parental intuition, observe the baby's reaction and, most importantly, put all your tenderness and love into the

movement of your hands. You can also use special massage oil. But avoid, as in the case of shampoo, strong-smelling products that can excite the baby, cause him to have allergies or breathing problems.

3. After the massage, put on your baby's pajamas. The procedure for putting on pajamas is perceived by most children as the first signal for sleep.

4. With the appearance of the first tooth in a baby, it is recommended that tooth brushing be part of the ritual. Then the baby will literally grow up with this habit, and brushing his teeth will be a matter of course for him. While the teeth are being formed and pushed out, the baby's gums are very sensitive, so you can use cotton swabs moistened with water to clean the first teeth. When the teeth will be a whole series, you can go to a special (small and soft) children's toothbrush.

5. Little children fall asleep better if the time before going to bed passes in a quiet, cozy

atmosphere with dim lights. Try to speak and sing softly. A cassette with a fairy tale or music should not sound too loud. If the child has to listen, he will make less noise and toss and turn in the crib.

6. It is better if the music is soothing and the tale is good. Exciting stories can excite the baby, and evil characters can cause dreams at night, disturbing his sleep. Many children quickly begin to nod if they read a fairy tale in a monotonous voice. Others with interest follow the course of events and love expressive reading, with a changing (depending on what character these words belong to) voice. It happens that a child likes a story so much that he asks to read (or tell) it every day. Thus, the child himself helps parents choose their evening ritual.

7. For older children, their own stories composed of parents reflecting, for example, the current situation in the family, have a great educational effect. So, in a naughty mouse, the baby will be able to recognize himself, and in a caring mother and mouse, his mother. A fairy tale

story will help the child to look at himself from the side and sometimes see the home situation in a completely new way. And the ability of kids to draw parallels is truly admirable!

8. Many children like falling asleep to lay next to their favorite toy, doll or even a rolled-up diaper, to which they can press their cheek. At that moment, your favorite soft toy or doll comes to life and becomes a faithful companion, to whom you can tell your joys and sorrows, which you can press harder to yourself so as not to feel lonely.

9. If the baby is afraid of the dark, you can leave the room, leave the nightlight turned on or stick special stars glowing in the dark on the ceiling of the children's room. One mother even came up with the custom of crafting special traps for fears with a child in the evening and put them in front of the door to the nursery. Well then, not a single bad dream and no fairy-tale characters dare to disturb the sleeping baby, right?

10. Children also like to talk or have a secret before going to bed with mom or dad. Especially in families where both parents work, for the baby this is often the only opportunity to stay face-to-face with parents, to share their feelings, concerns, ideas with them. And for parents, it's an opportunity to get to know their child closer: how he lives, how he develops, what he worries about ... Even if the baby spends all day with his mother, he is often so busy during the day with the game and what is happening around him that for intimacy, tenderness, and conversation it's simply not time remains. And in the evening, in peace and quiet, the whole atmosphere is conducive to affection and understanding. It is at the end of the day that a tired child needs them most.

11. The last minutes before bedtime is a wonderful chance to be with a child also for dad, who was at work all day. After all, the baby really needs dad's affection and care. And the proximity of dad at bedtime will allow the baby to fall asleep in the calm assurance that dad is nearby, loves him and will protect him all night.

12. With an older child, you can talk about the past day, remember pleasant events, and also tell him about plans for tomorrow. Children love when what is happening around them is understandable and predictable. Especially large, important events in children's life (trips, meetings with other people, holidays, etc.) require that the baby prepares for them, tune in to them. And even if we are talking about ordinary events (for example, about going to the store with mom), the child will be calmer and better behave there if you prepare him for this in advance and discuss the rules of behavior (stay near mom, do not scream, lack nothing without demand, etc.). You can also agree on what will happen if the baby does not follow these rules, just remember to fulfill the promise later, otherwise, the child will stop taking your words seriously!

13. A child who is already 3-4 years old and who has already learned to think, we can say that all his friends (it will be good to list them by name) have already gone to bed or are sleeping. Explain that this is the time when all the little children go to bed to gain strength for a new day. Recall that at this time he goes to bed every day and will go to bed further. As Allan Fromme, an American

psychologist and pediatrician, emphasizes in his book ABC for Parents, it is important that the child understands the need to go to bed, even if it contradicts his desire. Understanding that you cannot do only what we like in life will be the first important step on the path to the maturity of a little child.

14. You can tell the child that when you were little, you also went to bed at that time, and now you will be nearby to come to the baby if he calls you. And in the days when I was especially tired, I sometimes told my daughter that I went to bed and asked not to disturb me. Usually, she quietly fell silent in her crib and soon fell asleep peacefully.

15. Tell the child something good that he could think about, falling asleep, and wish him goodnight.

16. Arrange with the baby that in the morning, when he wakes up, he can come to your bedroom

and wake you up. This prospect helps many children fall asleep.

17. Sometimes I told my daughter: "Now I'll go clean the dishes in the kitchen (or wash in the bathroom, sew a hole in my trousers, cook soup, add a letter.) And then I will come to you again to wish you a good night. These words reassured my daughter, and when I looked again into her room, she was already sniffing quietly in her crib.

18. Older children like to fall asleep with an open or ajar door to the nursery (unless, of course, they are disturbed by the noise coming from other rooms). As soon as the baby falls asleep, the door can be closed. The arrangement with the child works very well: the door remains open, provided that he lies quietly in his crib. Most children do not like to stay behind a closed door, so they try to behave quietly and as a result fall asleep faster.

19. Often parents ask if the kids can watch TV at night. Of course, one good cartoon in the evening

will not hurt, but only one and only good. Scenes should not excite or frighten the child, which will interfere with his restful sleep. A TV should not be a substitute for parental attention. An evening cartoon can only be the starting point of the ritual, after which the baby begins to prepare for bed. But the child must spend the last minutes of the day with loved ones, in harmony and peace.

20. For older children, part of the ritual of falling asleep can be a quiet game alone in the children's room. We have already said that the older the baby becomes, the less sleep he needs and the later he falls asleep in the evening. But parents also need to rest in the evening hours. Therefore, a ritual combining the closeness of parents and independent play of the child in their room can be a good compromise.

21. For example, you can help your baby prepare for bedtime (brush his teeth, put on pajamas, etc.) and arrange with him that you will come to his room in half an hour or an hour. At this time, the child can (it always sounds more

attractive than "necessary") to stay in his room and play calmly. Usually, babies are happy to agree to this condition, if they are allowed to go to bed later. You can also show the child a watch and say that mom (or dad) will come to him when this arrow reaches this figure. As soon as the time is up, it is necessary to fulfill the promise, otherwise, the baby will stop believing in you.

22. If he, as promised, spent all his time playing calmly, then the second part of the ritual begins, in which the child has the undivided attention of his parents. This is a time of intimacy and tenderness, reading and music, conversation and secrets. This is a time of happiness for you and for your baby. Maybe he will wait for these minutes all day. Try and for a while, you forget about everything and plunge into the world of children's joy and imagination. After all, time passes very quickly. Do not have time to look around, as your chick will fly away from the nest, and you will regret with pain in your heart that you could not spend more time with him while he was little...

Even if you have not had the opportunity to engage with the baby all day, you can catch up during the evening ritual. Use these precious minutes for intimacy and affection, conversations, secrets, and calm games. It is these happy moments that will remain in the memory of the child for life!

Chapter 5: If the Child Does Not Want To Go To Bed Alone (Ferber Method)

But you introduced the ritual of falling asleep and a clear regimen, picked up the laying time when the child was really tired, and tried all the other tips given in this book, but your baby still refuses to fall asleep alone (and usually, as a result of this, he often wakes up at night).

What to do if your fatigue has reached the limit? What if you no longer have the strength to get up at night? What if in the evening you can no longer carry an incredibly tired creature that doesn't want to fit in a bed? In this case, you can, as a last resort, try out the method of the American professor Richard Ferber. As a doctor at a children's clinic in Boston, Richard Ferber founded a special center for the study of children's sleep. Ferber offers to consistently put the child in the crib alone while remaining nearby (for example, in the next room), and if the baby is crying, return to him at certain small intervals, comforting him, but not removing him from the crib. So, the baby will very quickly understand that he cannot achieve what he wants, and learns to fall asleep on his own.

Just do not listen to friends who recommend leaving the screaming child alone until he falls asleep. He will fall asleep - what else can he do if his long desperate calls for help go unanswered? (At a time when our grandparents were young, children were usually laid up like that, and they slept well all night.) But what happens in a small creature that nobody responds to crying? How does such a baby feel and what conclusions will he draw for himself for the future? He feels lonely, forgotten by all, and useless to anyone. He will put up with this and fall asleep, but the fear of loneliness and self-doubt will most likely remain for life. And if you can't stand it and after a long scream you still take the baby out of the crib, he will learn one more truth: "If you scream for a long enough time, I'll finally get my wish."

Therefore, for the successful application of the Ferber method, it is very important not to leave the crying child alone for a long time. Returning to the nursery at short intervals and comforting the baby with love, you will show him that you are nearby and love him, it's just the time for sleep, and he should fall asleep alone.

I repeat that the ideal option is, of course, to put the child to sleep without tears. The Ferber method is recommended only if for some reason you are unsuccessful and if you really have no more strength. After all, you know that the condition of the parents, especially the mother, is instantly transmitted to the baby. So, what is better - to carry baby on your hands day after day, falling from fatigue, or to withstand children's crying for several days, so that later, resting and getting enough sleep daily, you will happily devote yourself to the child? You decide. For those who want to try the Ferber method, I will try to describe it in more detail.

The following prerequisites are very important for success in using the Ferber method:

1. By the time you start using the method, the child must be older than 6 months and healthy.

2. In the coming weeks should not be any planned trips, overnight visits or other drastic

changes in the life of the baby. Until the new habit becomes permanent, the child should sleep at home in his crib. Changes in environmental conditions during the application of the method may interfere with the success of the enterprise.

3. But changing the place of sleep (for example, from the parents' bedroom to the children's room) just before you start following the method, on the contrary, can help the baby to acquire a new habit.

4. The kid should be accustomed to a certain regime and fall asleep at the same time. At the moment when you put the baby in the crib, he must be tired, his "internal clock" should already be switched to sleep.

5. You must be confident in your actions and ready to bring what you have started to the end.

6. An important prerequisite for applying this method is the unanimous decision of both parents.

Indeed, if mom puts the baby in the crib, and dad takes it out after 2 minutes (or vice versa), then, as you know, there will be no success.

Now in detail about the method:

Determine in advance at what intervals you will go to the baby to reassure him. Make an accurate plan that you will follow. The basic rule: for the first time, the wait time is a couple of minutes, then it gradually increases. When determining time intervals, rely on your intuition and do nothing against your inner voice. The waiting time can vary from 1 minute to half an hour.

It is best to start applying the method in the evening - at a time when the child usually falls asleep, or a little later. Spend the last minutes before bedtime with the baby, try to give him all your attention and tenderness at this time. It is very good if you already have an established evening ritual that the child is used to and which means for him to go to sleep.

Refuse this time from all the "helpers" who previously made it easier for the baby to fall asleep (bottle, chest, worn on the arms, motion in a stroller, etc.). All this should occur at least half an hour before bedtime. After the evening ritual, explain to the child that he is already large and must now learn to fall asleep on his own; then kiss him, put him in the crib, wish him goodnight and leave the room. When laying the baby, say the same phrase every day, for example: "And now, my dear, it's time to sleep." And leaving the room, you can, for example, say: "Goodnight! I love you very much!".

Since the child is not used to falling asleep alone, he will most likely begin to cry. In this case, proceed according to your plan and wait a few minutes before returning to his room. The plan begins with 3 minutes because usually, parents are not able to endure for the first time longer. But 3 minutes can seem incredibly long if you are standing outside the door and you hear the crying of your beloved child, so many prefer to start the wait from 1 minute. Be sure to look at the watch, because your own sense of time in these minutes stretches to incredibility.

If the baby is still crying, go into the room for a couple of minutes and try to calm him down without removing him from the crib. You can talk to the baby or pet him. Try to speak in a calm, firm voice, because the child will perfectly feel any insecurity in your actions. It is also important that the voice should sound without irritation and impatience, with love. Repeat again that it is time to sleep, that the baby is already big and must learn to fall asleep alone. Say mom is nearby and loves him. (Even if the baby still does not understand the words, he will feel warmth and love, as well as the confidence in your voice.) With these words, leave the room again, even if the baby is still crying. It is important that your stay in the room does not last too long. In no case should you give the baby bottles or pick them up.

If he gets up in the crib, lay him down before leaving the room (but only 1 time). Some children react to the appearance of their parents with an even more indignant scream. In this case, the stay of the parents in the room may be even shorter. But returning to the room at certain intervals is necessary so that the baby does not feel abandoned.

Leaving the room, follow the plan: wait for the time you set, then return to the nursery, repeating the previous steps, and so on until the baby falls asleep. If your presence in the room does not reassure the child, then the waiting time can be somewhat extended.

The next day, do the same, increasing only the number of minutes according to plan. The maximum waiting time (10 minutes) is better not to exceed. Come to the child only if he is really crying. A whimpering baby often calms down on its own. Therefore, in this case, it is better to wait a bit.

If the waiting periods seem very long to you, you can shorten them starting from 1 minute and not leaving the child alone for longer than 5 minutes. Even in this case, the above method will succeed.

Whatever plan you choose; the main thing is that you are able to implement it to the end. If you are bitten by doubts, choose the mildest option. However, only if you are confident in what you are doing, your actions will give the desired result. The child will feel your confidence and will not resist for long. For the same reason, it is not recommended to change the duration of waiting periods more than once. Frequent deviations from the plan will introduce uncertainty and unpredictability into your actions. Try to keep to one line. Knowing what to do next, you will feel calmer.

If you are afraid to leave the baby alone, then you can leave the room to talk with the child because from the closed or ajar door so he will be sure that you are nearby and did not leave him. Repeat that you love your baby, but that it's time to sleep, that he must learn to fall asleep in his bed alone, and tomorrow you will go for a walk with him ... (and further in the same vein).

Well, if this advice seems harsh to you, then you can stay in the room until the baby falls asleep. But act in this case according to the plan, approaching the baby only from time to time to console him. Then find the strength in yourself to move away and sit, say, on a chair away from the baby's bed, but so that he sees you. Pretend that you are reading or doing something (the light must be dim). If the child is crying, then at least you can be sure that he is crying not from fear, but simply because he does not receive what he wants. The main thing is for the baby to fall asleep on its own in its crib, without your help, without a bottle or other former "sleep helpers". Of course, in this case, you will need much more patience and time until he begins to fall asleep on his own. And if your presence in the room doesn't help and the baby cries every day anyway, then it's worth considering.

During the application of the method, it is very important to wake the child in the morning and afternoon at a time when he usually woke up – a little earlier. If the baby, falling asleep later than usual, has the opportunity to catch up this time later, then the entire regimen will be violated, and by the time of laying the child will not be tired enough. In this case, the self-falling asleep method will not work.

Mom and dad can succeed each other, putting the baby in the crib (but preferably not on the same night). The one who is more confident in the necessity of applying the method and who will be able to finish the job to the end should start.

Why Does the Ferber Method Work?

Accustomed to falling asleep with your help, the baby initially protests, ceasing to receive it. He screams, trying to scream to achieve what he wants. But what is going on? Mom or dad comfort him from time to time, however, not giving what he wants. The baby is terribly tired because in the morning he was woken up at an earlier time. "Is it worth shouting further," he thinks, "if all the same there is no use in this? I'm only wasting my energy, it's better to sleep just a little..." The need for sleep ultimately wins over the old habit that the kid wanted to restore.

As the waiting time for parents gradually increases, the baby understands that screaming longer is also useless. By this, he still will not get what he wants from his parents.

Falling asleep from fatigue day by day, the child gets used to falling into sleep on his own, this gradually becomes a habit. And the situation that has become habitual ceases to cause anxiety in the baby and replaces the old unfavorable habit in the subconscious.

When and How Often Should I Use the Ferber Method?

1. This method works best if you use it every time you go to bed, day and evening. But you can choose for a start only one time of the day, when the baby, in your opinion, is easier to fall asleep. Some children fall asleep easier on their own during the day. Many, especially older children, on the contrary, cannot be laid down during the day without the usual "helpers" to fall asleep.

2. If the baby does not fall asleep in the afternoon after 30 or 45 minutes, then do not to lay him at all and try to hold on to his next sleep time. In any case, this is better than giving him a bottle or what he is used to. Because then the baby will remember: "You cry for a long time - you will get what you wanted." There is no point in continuing attempts to lay the child, otherwise, his regimen will shift, and your nerves are unlikely to pass this test. Although holding out to the next time sleeping with a tired baby is also not so easy and requires great patience.

3. Well, if the baby fell asleep on the floor during the game, cover him with a blanket and let him sleep for half an hour. What no, but this is the first success - the child first fell asleep without your help.

4. If the baby's daytime sleep is very important to you, and without your help, he does not fall asleep during the day, then use the Ferber method at least in the evening. During the day, you use it when you can come to terms with the lack of a "quiet hour". The main thing is that, in principle, the baby learns to fall asleep alone, and the time of day at which he will do this can be gradually expanded.

5. For the speedy success of the Ferber method, use it also at night, when the baby wakes up. But, firstly, having learned to fall asleep on his own in the evening, the baby will most likely stop waking up at night on his own (more precisely, waking up at night, he will immediately fall asleep again without your help). Secondly, if the baby wakes up

at night, there is a danger that something hurts him or that he is scared of a terrible dream. In this case, he must be picked up and comforted. Thirdly, waking up at night, kids usually quickly fall asleep again. If the baby has to cry for a long time, this may disturb his sleep, and then he will not be able to fall asleep for a long time. And finally, I personally didn't have the strength to stand in front of the crying child's door at night. At night, I reassured my daughter in the usual ways. And having learned to fall asleep on her own in the evening, she simply stopped waking up at night!

6. If your baby falls asleep day and night alone, but still cries regularly at night, then it may be advisable to try the Ferber method at night.

7. Try to decide in advance what time you will use this method and which waiting periods you choose. I repeat that the predictability of further actions will facilitate the task for both you and the child.

What Problems Can Arise?

1. Some children are prone to vomiting and react to long cries. If vomiting occurs during the application of the self-falling asleep method, then go immediately to the baby, change his clothes, clean the room, change the bedding and follow the plan further, as provided. If you remain calm and confident, the child will quickly realize that vomiting does not affect your decision and learn to fall asleep on his own.

2. If one of the parents is unable to withstand the crying, he can go for a walk or put on headphones with music until the child falls asleep. You can even, to avoid unnecessary quarrels, use this method, for example, while your husband is on a business trip, and then surprise him with the finished results.

3. If the crib is in your room and you want the baby to fall asleep on his own also at night, then you can temporarily move the crib into another room or hang a curtain in front of it.

4. Brothers or sisters in the same room with the baby will also greatly complicate matters, and will also wake up from the crying of the youngest child. Try moving them temporarily to another room.

5. If the baby falls ill while following the Ferber method, then the application of the method must be interrupted. During illness, there can be no question of changing habits. When the child recovers, start all over again. This is also possible if the baby has already learned to fall asleep on his own, but due to his illness returned to old habits. You can return to the plan of self-falling asleep more than once, and each time the learning effect will be manifested faster.

Chapter 6: Temperament And Sleep: Understanding Your Child's Needs

Traditionally, science distinguishes four main types of temperament: sanguine, melancholic, phlegmatic and choleric. Each type of temperament has its own strengths and weaknesses, including, among other things, how the baby sleeps:

Sanguine people are cheerful and sociable, but it can be difficult to focus on one lesson, they are easily influenced by others, distracted. The transition from sleep to wakefulness and vice versa in these babies is quite easy, but external factors can distract their attention. During laying this can be expressed in the fact that the child does not want to switch to sleep - he jumps up, spins in bed, asks to eat, drink, play, etc. But, despite the fact that the child falls asleep for a long time, sanguine sleep is usually calm and consolidated.

The main features of choleric can considered activity and mild excitability. They are energetic, easily adaptable to changes, quickly "startup" and calm down for a long time, prone to irritability, it is difficult for them to maintain discipline. Parents of such babies often ask the question "How to lay it down?" Because they express their dissatisfaction loudly and violently, laying down can be delayed, the child falls asleep with tantrums, and sleep is often intermittent and restless.

Phlegmatic people are calm, persistent and stubborn. They love stability. The habits of phlegmatic people are formed for a long time and are very stable. In the usual circumstances, they calmly go to bed, quickly and firmly fall asleep, but changing conditions can unsettle them.

Melancholy - sensitive and impressionable. In response to changes in the environment and stressful situations tend to be offended, sad and locked in. Responsive, gentle and empathetic. They get tired quickly, so they fit relatively easily, but sleep can be disturbing. If a child often wakes up at night and cries without reasons such as physical discomfort or hunger, this is probably the effect of the melancholic type of temperament.

In its pure form, none of the types is practically not found, in any person, there are signs of each of them, mixed in different proportions. By the predominance of signs, each person belongs to a particular type of temperament.

The child's temperament is expressed in such characteristics as emotionality, ways of interacting with the surrounding reality, motor and speech activity, adaptability, etc. In order to better understand the possibilities and needs of your baby, it is worth considering these features and acting accordingly.

High Activity

There are hurricane children who run or jump, with a loud voice and a fast pace of speech, and there are calm and sedate babies who speak quietly, measuredly, or are completely silent, from which you won't get out a word and prefer to spend time browsing books or collecting puzzles. This does not mean that some can never be kept in place, while others cannot be "stirred up." They just have different needs for activity.

The organization of baby sleep requires attention in this matter. For calmer babies, to fall asleep, it is enough to wish goodnight and turn off the light, while active ones need a long gradual ritual to go into a sleepy state. Eating at bedtime can affect the activity of fidgets. Especially the feeding of "energy sweets". Therefore, if your baby in the evening begins to "stand on his head", it is worth moving the dinner to an earlier time and abandon the sweets for the night.

Sensitivity Level and Reaction Rate

Some babies, it seems, may wake up from a light breath, whispering or even looking in their direction, while others will not be bothered to sleep even by their neighbors' repairs or a dirty diaper. If your baby is sensitive, try to minimize the amount of irritants before laying. Carefully monitor the temperature in the bedroom, darken the room during sleep, if possible, keep silent (you can use white noise), make sure that vivid impressions and emotions occur mainly in the first half of the day, and spend evenings in the evening for quiet activities and keep calm yourself. Ensure that the laying conditions are as constant as possible so as not to cause undue concern.

Level of Focus and Distraction

Persistent children do not accept rejection. They are difficult to distract from the intended goal. And if this goal is to continue to stay awake when it's time to sleep, parents have to call on all their patience and willpower to help defeat the little stubborn.

To make laying easier, make the bedtime ritual as constant as possible. Try to strictly observe the time and procedure during the ritual every day.

Otherwise, if the child's attention is easily switched, it is worth removing all distracting factors from the sleep zone - lights, sounds, extra toys from the crib. The ritual should remain stable, and the conditions, as much as possible, unchanged.

Adaptability and Acceptance

An indicator related to the preceding paragraphs and expressed in how sensitive the child is to changing conditions. I note that, to one degree or another, changing conditions affect the sleep of each child, but some children adapt to new circumstances, whether it is changes in the ritual, moving to a new room (bed) or a long journey, quite quickly. To others, such innovations are given with great difficulty, causing problems with sleep and moods during laying. It is the level of sensitivity that determines how adaptive the child is to changes, and how much he will resist them. For example, the formation of a new habit requires 3 repetitions. For a sensitive baby, you may need 5.

To help sensitive children sleep better, try to approximate the conditions to the usual in emergency situations and observe them clearly in everyday life.

Rhythm

For some people, from childhood you can check the clock: they fall asleep, wake up and eat according to a clear internal schedule. It is about them that can be said: "War is war, and lunch is scheduled." When building a regime, this factor should be taken into account. Other children may forget about sleep and food if they are passionate about an interesting activity, or vice versa, upset or scared. It takes more time for such children to learn sleepy habits, but maintaining constant action will help them tune in to sleep at the right time.

Mood quality

Children prone to negative emotions, who are easily upset, also need stability more than eternal optimists. Such babies may feel sadness before going to bed with their mom, fear of the dark, it is difficult for them to cope with their experiences.

More sensitive physical interactions should be included in the ritual for sensitive children. Hugs, kisses, stroking, light massage will help them to relax and feel more confident. Sensitive toys come in handy. A soft toy will provide tactile sensations and help to cope with loneliness. If the child is afraid to fall asleep in the dark, for the time of falling asleep, you can leave the dim nightlight on.

The skill of independent falling asleep and the continuity of night sleep are directly dependent on temperament, so you need to understand your child and adapt his (or her) needs to your ritual routines.

The individual characteristics of temperament do not make one child better than another. It is they who make up his unique personality. They affect all spheres of life; therefore, our task is to help our kids use their potential as efficiently as possible. High-quality rest is one of our main allies, and the main tools that help us in establishing full sleep are stability and a regime based on understanding the individual needs of the child. Watch the reactions of your baby, and then the answer to the question of how to put the baby to bed will become more obvious.

Different Results for Different Temperaments

When will the first successes be noticeable? Of course, it depends on the temperament of the child, on the energy with which he resists the new circumstances and what "lessons" he had to "learn" in his still very short life.

The first days will, in any case, be a test for both you and the baby. But some children do not cry for more than 15 minutes and after 2-3 days fall asleep in the crib on their own. Others cannot calm down at first for an hour or two, and parents have to go into their room ten times or more often with the words: "I am here, I love you, but you have to go to sleep. You are already big and should fall asleep alone in your crib."

However, if you patiently and consistently apply your plan, you can expect the first improvement, and sometimes even the solution, on the third day. After all, children learn much faster than adults and can quickly adapt to new situations.

Some kids take a little longer. But the acquisition of a new habit rarely lasts longer than a week, and only in some cases longer than two weeks. After your baby has managed to fall asleep ten times in a row on his own, you can assume that the most difficult is behind! You can sit back and relieve a sigh of relief.

Forget about dirty laundry for a while, leave the iron and mop alone. Give yourself a few minutes - a hot bath, a walk or a run, a delicious dinner, your favorite music. Restore your strength, raise your mood, and then any work will take much less time. And a look at the peacefully sleeping baby will fill you with the consciousness that a new era has come, in which there is also room for your desires and interests!

Chapter 7: Children's Fears and Sleep Disorders for Other Reasons

A baby can wake up at night not only due to a natural change in the phases of sleep, erupting tooth, or a cold that begins. Sometimes night awakenings can be associated with other reasons, for example: trembling in a dream, interruptions in a baby's breathing (sleep apnea), incomplete awakening from deep sleep (sleepwalking and nightly fright), fears, problems and nightmares that torment a child, etc. On each of these phenomena, you will find special medical literature or might need to consult a doctor, so we will only touch on these topics briefly, talking about the most important things.

Jerking in a dream

Sometimes the baby wakes up because he trembles in a dream or when falling asleep. At these moments, individual muscle groups are unevenly tensed and relaxed. The reason may be overexcitation before bedtime, as well as loud sounds that frighten the baby. Do not be alarmed or make sudden movements. Most likely, the baby, having opened his eyes and making sure that everything is in order, will again fall into a nap.

If the startles are repeated several times in a row and have no apparent reason, then we can talk about convulsions. In this case, you must definitely show the child to a pediatric neurologist.

Breaks in breathing (sleep apnea)

Some children suddenly begin to snore in a dream without being caught a cold. If you listen carefully, then snoring is interrupted from time to time, and the baby does not breathe for some time (up to 10 seconds). This phenomenon is called sleep apnea and is due to the fact that the flow of air along the way into the trachea is interrupted. Sometimes the muscles of the throat relax during sleep so much that the tongue falls back and blocks the flow of air. Enlarged glands and adenoids are also a common cause. In the afternoon, these children often seem sleepy and tired. Sometimes, on the contrary, they are overly active, or parents notice any other changes in their behavior.

If you notice signs of sleep apnea in your child, you should definitely show it to your doctor. In most cases, enlarged glands or adenoids have to be removed, but the baby again sleeps soundly and calmly at night.

Narcolepsy: mystic illness

An unusual disease in which a person is not able to control his own sleep and wakefulness is called "narcolepsy." It came from the Greek words narkē, meaning numbness, and lēpsis - dream.

Narcolepsy is a fairly rare disease (out of 2 thousand affects 1 person). It develops mainly in 20-50-year-old men, but it can also appear in childhood. Despite the low prevalence, this pathology is very dangerous, because the individual can suddenly fall asleep at anytime and anywhere, performing some kind of action. Such an attack is not subject to control; therefore, it is an obstacle to normal activity. Children with such a disease usually lag behind in development. The feelings of narcolepsy are similar to those experienced by people who have not slept for two days, and this reduces the quality of life. Researchers cannot explain the exact cause of the drowsiness syndrome since it has not been studied enough due to its uniqueness. However, it turned out that psychological and psychiatric problems are not to blame. Currently called such factors for the development of the disease:

- heredity;
- lack of special genes for hypocretins (orexins) - neurotransmitters that provide signaling to sleep and waking in the brain;
- impaired immune system;
- severe infections;
- skull injuries;
- viral diseases;
- malfunctions of the endocrine glands, including the pituitary gland.

This causes a strong desire to sleep during the day, despite a sufficient amount of night sleep. Such irresistible drowsiness interferes with normal activity, as it is accompanied by lethargy, nebulous thinking, apathy, difficulty concentrating. The baby feels "broken", "squeezed like a lemon", constantly tired. He has no mood, he is constantly irritated, cannot remember important information, and loses motivation. At any time and under any circumstances, the child may fall asleep, and such attacks occur several times a day. It is easy to wake him up and after waking up he, just for a while, feels rested.

Unfortunately, it is impossible to completely get rid of this neurological disorder, but it is quite possible to correct and thereby improve the quality of life.

Head Banging

This may sound surprising, but intentional head banging is extremely common among babies. According to statistics, 20 percent of babies especially bang their heads, while boys among them are three times as many girls. According to experts, for the first time, a child tries to bang his head in the second half of the first year of life. Peaks of head-hitting occur in 18-24 months. The vast majority of children outgrow this problem by the age of three, but for some, it continues even at school.

The reasons why the child bangs his head are as follows:

1. Personal comfort. No matter how strange it sounds, the lion's share of children 2-4 years old resorts to head bangs to ... relax. Head bangs are a rhythmic movement, and such ones just soothe the baby. Therefore, the child beats his head.

2. The pain. The child deliberately bangs his head even when he experiences pain elsewhere (as an option - a toothache). A deliberate knock on the head and the discomfort caused by this distracts the baby from that pain.

3. A way out of emotions. Young children still do not know how to express feelings in any other way than physical actions. Even if the baby already knows how to speak, he does not resort to the help

of words to indicate his own feelings. And therefore, during tantrums, in order to give vent to strong emotions, the child beats his head. Here, in addition, the "two in one" principle works: the baby expresses emotions and consoles itself during stress.

4. Attraction of attention. Children are much smarter and more insightful than we think. If the baby does not have enough attention from the side of mom and/or dad, but he noticed that they flap wings over him when he hits, the child will resort to blows with his head - so parents will definitely pay attention to him.

5. Another reason why the child bangs his head lies in the problems of the development of the child (autism and other disorders), but this rarely happens, in the vast majority of cases, the child bangs his head for the other reasons described above.

How to Deal with It

1. Pay attention to the baby. Not when the child bangs his head, but at other times. Play with the baby, talk, walk - behave like a standard loving parent. After all, are you like that?

2. Do not attach importance, otherwise, the child is able to beat his head even harder. It is impossible to ignore - at least do not scream, do not scold and do not punish.

3. Limit your child's access to hard surfaces. Move the crib away from the wall, hang the sides of the cradle cushions, and so on.

4. Do not worry. Yes, a child can bump slightly and make a bruise. But a header is a self-regulating phenomenon, the baby is unlikely to cause serious injury to himself. He knows the threshold of his own pain and will die of ardor as needed.

5. Show your baby other ways to express rhythm. A header is partly attractive to the child because it is rhythmic. But other things are also rhythmic: dance, marching, drumming and so on.

6. Provide your child with outdoor games so that he burns the nervous energy that makes him bang his head.

7. If the child bangs his head before bedtime, enter a relaxing and calming ritual - a warm bath, massage, soft music or reading, a glass of milk and so on.

8. If the child beats his head constantly throughout the day and does not stop, even hurting himself, consult a doctor. Pay attention to other features in the behavior of the baby. If the child is not interested in contact with people, including parents; looking not at a person, but as if through him; loses acquired skills / physical abilities; turns into a closed and detached - these are signs of the

development of autism. In this case, a doctor's consultation is required.

Nighttime Incontinence - Bed Wetting

Nighttime incontinence occurs when a child pees while sleeping without realizing it. Many children go to the bathroom without problems during the day-long before being clean all night. Indeed, it takes sometimes several months, if not several years, before a child is clean all night.

Most, but not all children stop wetting their beds between 5 and 6 years old. Nighttime incontinence is more common in boys and children who have a deep sleep.

What Is the Cause of Nocturnal Incontinence?

Most of the time, nocturnal incontinence is related to deep sleep. The child's bladder is full, but he does not wake up. Some children have a small bladder or produce more urine during the night. Constipation can also cause nighttime incontinence because the bowel presses on the bladder.

If your child has always wet their bed and has never spent the night dry for at least 6 months, he has no particular problem. This type of nocturnal incontinence is not caused by medical, emotional or behavioral problems.

However, if your child has been dry all night for at least 6 months and is starting to get wet again, talk to your doctor.

Should We Cure Nocturnal Incontinence?

In general, no. It is important to ask yourself if night incontinence disturbs your child. If she does not mind, you probably do not need to have it treated. The problem eventually settles itself in most children.

What Else Can I Do to Help My Child?

1. Make sure your child does not drink too much before going to bed.
2. Avoid drinks that contain caffeine (such as soft drinks).
3. Encourage your child to go to the bathroom before going to bed.
4. Wear training pants or diapers.
5. Cover the mattress with a plastic cover designed for hospitals to prevent damage to the mattress.
6. Place a large towel under the sheet to promote additional absorption.
7. It is not necessary to wake a sleeping child who has wet his bed. There is no harm to sleeping in wet sheets. It is more important for everyone to enjoy a good night's sleep.
8. Do not wake your child to go peeing when already bed. You will not solve his incontinence, but you will disturb his sleep.
9. When your child wets his bed, help him wash well in the morning so that he does not feel bad.

When Should I Talk to My Doctor?

Consult your doctor and if your child:

- has been clean several months, then suddenly starts to wet his bed.
- has other symptoms, such as a burning sensation when urinating.

Cri-du-chat: The Cry Baby Syndrome

The cri du chat command, or cat cry syndrome, is a rare genetic disease. Symptoms of the disease include numerous body distortions, especially noticeable on the face. A characteristic symptom of cat cry disease is the creaky scream of a baby, reminiscent of a cat's call. The most characteristic drawback is the delay or complete lack of speech development. Kids with cri du chats start talking late.

One of the first observed features of a baby from a cry baby syndrome is low birth weight and decreased muscle tone. However, it should be remembered that these are nonspecific symptoms and can occur for various reasons. A very common and important symptom is a shrill and monotonous baby crying like a cat is wandering. This is due to the wrong design of the larynx, and the fold that closes the entrance to it, i.e. epiglottis.

In small patients, this includes, but is not limited to: microcephaly - the perimeter of the baby's head is disproportionately small, round-like a moon face, hypertelorism - the wide distance of the eyeballs, outstanding frontal tumors, short and wide base of nose, which enhances the impression of wide divergence of eyes, distorted and low set ears

- bone distortion, etc.

The diagnosis of a "cry baby" is mainly based on clinical observations - a baby with low birth weight and a characteristic cry. A physician may order a karyotype to confirm for the deletion of the short arm of chromosome 5.

With the proper help of specialists, you can avoid or reduce the inconvenience caused by the disease. As the baby grows, the face could also change.

Growing Teeth

If some babies have their first teeth without any hassle, others suffer a lot. What will you see in a baby before a new tooth?

Red and swollen gums, an excess of drool, a disturbed sleep, a drop in appetite, a grouchy state often accompanies the dental surges of babies. Some parents notice that their child has a fever or diarrhea just before a tooth pierces.

Treat each symptom individually and consult your doctor or pediatrician if you are worried. You may also notice that your baby has redness on the chin or lower lip, drooling. Gently wipe the slime with a clean cloth or cotton, without rubbing. You can also apply a soothing cream before bedtime to relieve the irritation.

What Are the Solutions to Calm the Dental Pain?

The teeth of your baby started their development while you were pregnant: tooth buds have formed in the gums. As the teeth grow, they press against the gums, causing irritation, pain, and swelling.

Gently putting your finger on your sore gums can temporarily calm the pain. Give him an object to bite: the pressure on the gums will soothe his pain.

There is a good chance your baby is biting himself whatever comes to hand. Hard pieces, such as raw carrots, or a teething ring can help. Cold items also have a soothing virtue. Keep teething rings cool. Offer him a small towel or washcloth passed through the ice cube compartment, and he can chew. To calm the gums, freshwater in a bottle can help. If the baby is already used to solid foods, offer him yogurts or compotes very cold.

Sometimes your baby will refuse anything you try to give him. A hug will be the best way to console his misfortunes.

Can I Use Anesthetic Gels and Homeopathy?

A little soothing gel rubbed on the sore baby's gum, with a clean finger, helps to anesthetize the pain for a moment. Nevertheless, do not apply gel more than 6 times a day. If you are breastfeeding, take care not to breastfeed. The gel can indeed anesthetize the baby's tongue which can prevent sucking properly. The gel could also lull your areola (dark skin around the nipple), making feeding more difficult. You can also try homeopathic granules, available in pharmacies. These are tiny balls that you can let melt in your baby's mouth.

Can I Give Paracetamol to My Baby?

If all else fails, and you and your baby are really disarmed by these dental surges, you can give him paracetamol. Of course, take the doses prescribed by your doctor or pharmacist. First, make sure that the baby does not cry for another reason. Otitis is often confused with simple dental flare. If your child has a temperature, consult your doctor.

How Long Will the Dental Flares Last?

Just as it is impossible to predict when a baby's first tooth will appear, no one can know how long the flare-ups will last. Some babies will only be bothered for a few days before a tooth pierces. Others will have several unpleasant symptoms for months without any breakthrough!

The good news is that for most babies, the first teeth are the hardest to get out. The discomforts associated with a new tooth sometimes persist until the arrival of molars, the teeth in the back of the mouth is towards baby's first birthday.

Food Refluxes

According to one study, about 24% of infants suffer from gastro-oesophageal reflux, causing regurgitation after meals and sometimes severe pain in the baby. Without significant consequences in most cases, complicated GERD can be said to cause significant discomfort for the child and, in rare cases act on the growth of the child and the well-being of the whole family.

GERD, diminutive of the term "gastroesophageal reflux", commonly called food reflux, is a rise in the contents of the stomach in the baby's esophagus.

This rise is due, among other things, to the fact that the junction between the esophagus and the stomach, called cardia, which has for initial purpose to prevent the rise of the gastric contents, did not finish its formation.

Attention, GERD is not to be confused with the simple rejection due to too much food. Indeed, a baby who has eaten a bit too much will spit the overflow in the corner of the lips very quickly after the meal, while the GERD is characterized by lifts that can last for several hours and potentially painful given the acidity that accompanies these lifts.

How Do You Know That Your Child Has GERD?

There are several symptoms that can alert you. In the simplest cases, it will be:

- Low or more abundant regurgitation between meals.
- Sleep problems due to acidity that makes baby uncomfortable.

In more severe cases, this may also result in vomiting, repeated bronchitis or frequent sore throat or ear infections, discomfort such as choking, and severe stunting in severe cases.

How to Relieve Baby?

In the case of GERD, there are some tips that can immediately and easily relieve baby. Here are a few tips:

- First of all, never leave your baby flat on your back: use an incline so that it is positioned at a constant 30 to 40 degrees to the mattress.
- During meals, make sure that the baby does not eat too quickly.
- Once the meal is over, keep the baby in the upright position. So, keep it in your arms or use a carrier if you are busy.

- If you are not breastfeeding, use thicker anti-regurgitation milk than traditional milk. Also, be sure to use a slow flow nipple.
- In all cases of GERD, it is important to talk to your pediatrician. For more severe cases of reflux, medical treatments are prescribed to small patients.

GERD, A Temporary Evil

Although not to be taken lightly, know that GERD is a temporary ailment. Indeed, GERD declines as soon as the baby diversifies his food and muscles his abdomen and when the child is sitting. This evil will also tend to disappear with the acquisition of walking.

Sleepwalking

You already know that the baby's deep sleep phase is interrupted from time to time by moments of incomplete awakening. Usually, these moments go unnoticed. The child, perhaps, flips over to another side, mutters something, opens his eyes for a short moment, and without any problems again plunges into a deep sleep. But sometimes children linger in a similar state of being half-awake. At this time, they can talk, walk and perform other unconscious movements and actions (sleepwalking), as well as scaredly screaming, not realizing this and not responding to your presence (nightly fright).

Do not be alarmed - in most cases this condition is not dangerous, and until the age of six, it is usually not associated with mental disorders, nor with fears or problems. According to doctors, the predisposition to sleepwalking is transmitted genetically and is associated with many children with the process of brain formation.

If your baby in this condition moves around the room, then you must make sure that he cannot get hurt, open a window or front door, go out to the balcony, etc.

In addition, he must necessarily get enough sleep at night and not get too tired during the day (tired children sleep especially deeply). Therefore, try to adhere to a clear daily routine.

Night Fright

If a child suddenly screams or cries in the first 3-4 hours after falling asleep (sometimes it also waves its arms, sweats, and its heart beats faster) and does not allow you to come to it, then it is in a state of nightly fright. He sees a terrible dream but does not wake up from it. Do not try to wake the baby at this moment. Make sure that he is not injured. Do not panic. In the morning - the child will not be able to remember anything. An attack of nightly fright can quickly pass, but it can last up to 20 (or even 30) minutes. Then the child suddenly calms down, relaxes and peacefully falls asleep. Over time, the night's fright goes away on its own, so reassure yourself with the thought that this phenomenon is temporary and not dangerous.

Especially often nightmares torment children in the period from 3 to 6 years. At this age, the child already sees and knows a lot, but still does not understand everything. He still does not have life experience, so he may be afraid of a new and unfamiliar, frightening events and unexpected situations. A quarrel between parents, a big dog suddenly arising in front of a child, a car braking sharply, a frightening-looking passerby who spoke to the baby - everything that made a strong impression on him or frightened him during the day can be reflected in frightening dreams.

The border between the real idea of the world and the fantasy of young children is still very vague, and often children are afraid of their own inventions. Fantasies suddenly start to get out of hand, become naughty and scary. Ghosts, trolls and other fairy-tale figures or cartoon characters begin to haunt the baby, creep up to his crib and disturb his nightly calm.

Very often, children are afraid of the dark. Usually, this is a fear acquired - either inspired by us, or that arose after an event that frightened the child. Tales and films reinforce this fear, populating night time with all kinds of spirits, demons, vampires and other evil spirits.

Newborn babies are scared of harsh sounds and large objects approaching them. They worry in the absence of a mother, and from 7-8 months they begin to fear unfamiliar adults.

If you punish a child, then he may be tormented by the fear of punishment, also reflected in nightmares.

Conflicts in the family almost always lead to childhood fears and problems. Kids who often watch TV may be afraid of the events they saw there, such as fire, war, the elements, attack, fight, etc. Fears appear in children after surgery, a serious illness, or the death of someone in the family.

Sometimes parents bully kids, without thinking about the consequences. "If you don't obey, you will be taken by an uncle a policeman", "Don't make noise, otherwise ghost granny will come", "You'll reach, otherwise a terrible bear will take you to the forest" - parents don't resort to such scary "masterpieces" to act to your child. If the baby believes you, this is terrible. So, you, the only close and beloved people, agree to give it to ghost granny or the bear because of the half-eaten porridge? Who, besides you, will protect him? Left alone with his fear, the baby will surely be afraid of the dark and suffer from nightmares. Well, if he didn't believe you, he never once met ghost granny, he didn't see a terrible bear except in the zoo, and the uncle doesn't care about his whims, then the baby will be convinced that you lie to him to make him obedient. He will learn for himself that you can lie, and that's fine. Did you want to achieve this?

Often fears in babies and young kids are by overly patronized parents. "Beware - you will fall!", "Do not touch the dog - it will bite!", "Do not go - you will get hit!", "Get dressed - you will catch a cold!" of the dangers alone, which he, so small and weak, cannot resist!

It is especially difficult for kids who have anxious, fearful parents. They convey their fear to the child, and this is truly a difficult test for the child's psyche.

What to Do If Your Child Has Fears?

First, stop scaring the baby and being scared yourself! Find out the cause of fear. Treat fear with understanding, never scold or shame your baby for him.

Assure that you will always protect him. Help your child overcome fear by playing, drawing, and playing frightening situations.

If the baby is afraid of the dark, leave the nightlight on. Never lock your child in a dark room.

If he is afraid of fairy-tale heroes, try to turn them from evil to good (for example, Grandma Hedgehog can suddenly become good grandfather and grandmother, and a terrible bear can turn into a little shaggy little bear). Do not read more tales with scary characters.

Watch your baby watching TV. Avoid frightening and aggressive gears.

A toy weapon lying at night next to his crib can comfort a boy. It will help him repel imaginary enemies if they only dare to approach him at night.

Do not try to convince the child with words, because he still cannot control his emotions.

Increase the baby's self-esteem, praise him, promote the development of his independence.

Well, finally, deal with your own fears and problems, because it is they who most often "infect" our children!

Chapter 8: The Father's Role in Comforting Children

Whether the parental couple is united or not, the role of the father remains fundamental in the construction of the child, from birth to adulthood. May dad take his place!

Sometimes he is there for the birth, but sometimes he tends to leave the mother, alone, in the face of education and especially in the face of the trials of growth.

In the mind of your child, a good image of the father will play its role satisfactorily. Greater participation in care from an early age facilitates the early recognition of a good image of the father. At age 6, if the integrated image until now is good enough, the father is perceived on a mode of fascination "my dad is the most beautiful, the strongest", but it is in adolescence, if it has poorly preserved, that the good image of the father is most likely to be questioned.

The Father Helps to Build the Personality of His Child

The role of the father is different from that of the mother and is complementary. From the earliest ages, the father provokes a faster awakening, more open sociability, and a more precocious control of language, etc. Schematically, mom comforts, daddy stimulates.

The father participates in the construction of the child's personality by promoting the acquisition of the autonomy and independence necessary for a balanced emotional life and the self-confidence useful in future competitions. In this role, he prevents the mother from being an abusive mother by helping her to accept that her child will eventually be separated from her. It is sometimes difficult because mothers tend to monopolize the place, but new fathers from this point of view change the situation, provided that at some point they are not caught up in their work.

The absence of the father can cause an imbalance in your child. The father's absences may arise from professional reasons, death, illness, lack of interest in family life, non-recognition of the child, but most often of a court decision related to a divorce or separation.

When separating the parents, it is essential that the father retains his role of educator whatever the circumstances. If the father dies, then the male entourage becomes important. If, on the other hand, the father's image deteriorates, your child may feel insecure and may compensate for his relationship with the mother.

If you cannot respond to this situation, your child may become anxious and unstable. Ideally, a father encourages his child to excel, to oppose him in competition. In this process, your child becomes autonomous and independent.

Alterations in the paternal image lead to identification difficulties for the child, difficulties in his communication skills, fostering inhibition, instability, a tendency to doubt himself and to devalue himself. These children are often depressed.

In conclusion, if the paternal image is abused, your child may have character disorders. It can become unstable, aggressive, hyper-emotional, anxious, impulsive, enclosed or excited, in short, trouble begins.

Therefore, involve dad in the development of his child. Encourage them to do activities, between them, it gives you time for you. Whether it's a girl or a boy, let them form a winning duo. In case of separation, encourage dads and children to see each other regularly, except in extreme danger.

In short, you two conceived this child, the sleep and basic education must be done by two, at least until adulthood.

Conclusion

I conclude this book by mentioning a few "hacks" that you have probably considered. Should the baby just sleep on my bed? Great idea, that way, you must have skipped most of the hard work, right?

Well, experts say that even if from the first days of life a newborn sleeps with his mother, he should have a crib. It can be left in it during the day, especially when he has already learned to roll over, crawl. A woman cannot fully relax when her baby is nearby. In this matter, doctors advocate reasonable flexibility.

In any case, research shows that staying children at night in spouses' bed often causes divorces in many families. Returning from the hospital, a woman gives herself completely to the child, but not every man is able to bear it. The marital bed remains the only place where the husband can claim the care of his wife, so the presence of the baby causes extreme discontent.

Can medicines help baby sleep? Here's number two. Well, as you most likely should know, sleeping pills, sedatives and other medicines are just short-term help, fraught with dangerous consequences! The child will fall asleep at the moment, but the cause of poor sleep will not be eliminated. Therefore, as soon as the medication is stopped, all problems with falling asleep and sleeping at night will come back. In addition, potent drugs have many side effects that are extremely dangerous for a young, not yet fully formed organism. From taking medication, if the child is healthy, you must completely refuse.

Try the simple remedies proposed in this book. They are tried and trusted and you will reap decent dividends in no time at all!

Finally, if you found this book useful in any way, a review on Amazon is always appreciated!

www.ingramcontent.com/pod-product-compliance
Lightning Source LLC
Chambersburg PA
CBHW072024230526
45466CB00019B/383